THE JUICE

MADE EASY

WITH TIPS, TRICKS & HEALTHY FRUIT & VEGETABLE JUICE RECIPES.

JEM FRIAR N.C.

THE PERSONAL DETOX COACH

THE PERSONAL DETOX COACH'S SIMPLE GUIDE TO HEALTHY LIVING SERIES

COPYRIGHT

PUBLISHERS NOTES

Disclaimer

This publication is intended to provide helpful and informative material. It is not intended to diagnose, treat, cure, or prevent any health problem or condition, nor is intended to replace the advice of a physician. No action should be taken solely on the contents of this book. Always consult your physician or qualified health-care professional on any matters regarding your health and before adopting any suggestions in this book or drawing inferences from it.

The author and publisher specifically disclaim all responsibility for any liability, loss or risk, personal or otherwise, which is incurred as a consequence, directly or indirectly, from the use or application of any contents of this book.

Any and all product names referenced within this book are the trademarks of their respective owners. None of these owners have sponsored, authorized, endorsed, or approved this book.

Always read all information provided by the manufacturers' product labels before using their products. The author and publisher are not responsible for claims made by manufacturers.

Print Edition 2015

Manufactured in the United States of America

A Gift To Help You With Your Juicing

In appreciation for you buying this book and to help you with your new juicing habit I would like to give you a quick reference guide to preparing any and all of the fruits and vegetables that you might want and need to put in your juicer.

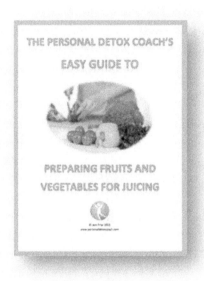

I will also inform you about any updates to this kindle book (more tips and recipes) or other juicing and health books in the Personal Detox Coach's Simple Guide to Healthy Living Series as they are released, as well as occasionally send you more scrumptious juice recipes to keep you inspired.

To get your free guide, your tips, more juice recipes and your updates go to:
http://www.personaldetoxcoach.com/JuiceHabitBookSign

WHY I WROTE THIS BOOK

I wrote this book because after working with thousands of people in the world of juicing and detox retreats since 2000, I have learnt 2 very clear things:

- Juicing regularly can create a phenomenal amount of health benefits and help promote many positive changes in a person's life.

- People often struggle to make the simple changes and adopt the beneficial habits that would make regular juicing (and it's many benefits) part of their lives.

It seems a tragedy that not more people adopt this very simple habit and maintain it. I felt that by writing this book to show how and why to juice, to provide some delicious and mouth watering juice recipes but most importantly to provide lots of helpful tips and tricks to make regular juicing easier, it will support many more people to adopt and keep up this great habit.

I am trained in Naturopathy and I have specialised in running traditional juice fasts and detoxes since the turn of the 21st century. Many of the juice books that are available dismay me because often the recipes contain ingredients that are not healthy or helpful e.g. sugar, alcohol, milk. Some of these recipes contain grains, bananas or avocado, and although these are healthy, to me they are no longer pure juices but rather smoothies. My approach is that if it is not a fruit or vegetable or if it wont go through a juicer and come out from the juice spout (as opposed to the pulp collector), then it is not a real juice.

Juicing has become a lot more popular in recent years and in fact is presently rather trendy. The fact that juicing is now often mentioned on TV and in the media is great. Many extremely healthy looking celebrities are keen on extoling the value of their daily juice regime. There are also many stories about people healing themselves from long standing chronic diseases by taking up daily juicing. All of these inspirations have encouraged hundreds of thousands of people to take up the juicing habit or to buy a juicer.

I have met and worked with many, many people who already own their own juicer, which is great but not necessarily enough. You have to use it too!

It is quite remarkable how many people's juicers are buried in an obscure cupboard or are collecting dust on a hard to get to, top shelf. So why is it that such a quick and easy way to boost your nutrient intake, get healthier and feel fantastic, becomes forgotten, neglected or is even never tried in the first place? We will look at that in this book but more importantly, I will give you tried and tested tips and suggestions for getting out of such a predicament and to help you become enthusiastic about an easy process of regular juicing.

It is actually possible to use specific juices or fruits and vegetable to help overcome certain illnesses, however, in this book I have not gone into any detail about which juices are useful for what illnesses. There are other books in this series that go more specifically into which juices, fruits and vegetables might be most helpful for specific imbalances. In this book my intention is to inspire you to drink a mixed variety of juices regularly, as this will be incredibly useful for boosting your health and immunity in general.

I have written this book in a simple style because I know that people live in a busy world and don't necessarily have time to lounge around reading on a sofa for a few days just to get to grips with a subject. My suggestions and tips are not complicated or difficult. I am a firm advocate of simplicity as this path offers the most effective results. My motto is "keep it simple, keep it smart".

In a similar way, I have not included hundreds of juice recipes that might provide you with so much choice that you don't actually choose any. I would rather make your choosing easy and also encourage you to start experimenting and creating your own juices too.

There is an overwhelming amount of information that is available to us in books, videos and on the internet. I see no reason to overburden your mind with even more unnecessary information and things to do. My goal was to create a book that clearly summarizes all of the important aspects of juicing, whilst also provide easily actionable tips to allow people to become "Juicers" effortlessly.

Jem Friar

www.personaldetoxcoach.com

WHY YOU SHOULD READ THIS BOOK

It can be very challenging to adopt healthier habits into our lives because we often think that doing so will be hard work. Using my own experience and the helpful experiences of the thousands of people that I have worked with, I am providing you with suggestions and information that can make adopting juicing as a lifestyle quick and painless.

This book will help you to find an easy way to incorporate regular juicing in your life by showing you:

Why juicing is so beneficial

How to juice in an effortless way

How to avoid the pitfalls that often stop people from juicing regularly

And it will also give you some fabulous recipes which you can explore and use.

You should also read this book because it will be simple to follow and therefore the ideas and tips will be easy to incorporate into your life.

If you have children who you would love to be enjoying fresh juices with you, then there is also a short chapter of tips that particularly relate to inspiring kids.

To really make juicing an easy and enjoyable routine I encourage you to read chapter 4 "Tips and Tricks To Make Regular Juicing Much Easier" before you begin juicing and then go back and read through the headings several times as you are getting in to your juicing habit.

There is an incredible amount of evidence about the health benefits of increasing our intake of fruits and vegetables, such as reducing the risk of heart disease, cancer, diabetes, etc. Drinking freshly made juices has got to be the easiest and most efficient way of massively increasing our fruit and veg intake.

And beyond these reasons – fresh juices taste great and will make you feel awesome!

Regular juicing can have a profound, positive impact on your health and wellbeing, so I heartily encourage you to try it out.

I wish you a long, healthy, vibrant and joyful life.

TABLE OF CONTENTS

CHAPTER 1. WHAT IS SO GREAT ABOUT JUICING?

People get into fresh juices for many reasons: they taste great, it is trendy; they want to lose weight, they want to get healthy, they want to stay healthy, their friends are always drinking juices, a celebrity is always drinking juices etc.

Being clear why you yourself have become interested in drinking more fresh juices is a really important question to answer because this clarity will help you take on board this information and these suggestions.

So before I go any further, take a minute to ask yourself why you are interested in knowing more about the value of fresh juicing and how you can juice more often. Write it down if it helps.

*****

I hope that you have asked yourself and are now clearer as to why you specifically want to know more about juicing (and if you haven't, then stop reading and ask yourself now). You will find it really helpful to have this clarity as a starting point.

In this chapter I will give you lots of other great reasons which will hopefully inspire you even more to adopt a regular fresh juicing lifestyle.

WHAT IS A JUICE?

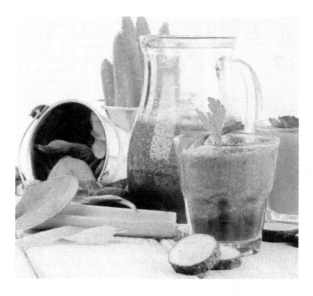

Firstly, I would like to clarify what I mean by a fresh juice, as juice means lots of different things to many people.

When I am talking about juices, I mean ones that have just been extracted with a juicer from fresh fruits and vegetables by you (or perhaps by someone in a great juice bar, if you are out). When making a pure juice, you will only really have one main piece of kitchen equipment to clean afterwards – your juicer – which keeps the juicing process easy and quick.

I am not referring to juices that are found in cartons and bottles in shops and supermarkets. These are overly processed and lack vitamins, nutrients and life force. Many have various additives and sweeteners. They are also often full of sugar, which is definitely something that you would do well to be removing from your diet.

There are also some blenders that purport to make fresh juices like the Vitamix or the Nutribullet. Whilst both of these machines are great and very useful, neither of them create what I would describe as real juices. They actually make vegetable and/or fruit smoothies because the juice is not extracted from the mass of the fruits and/or vegetables and the fiber is left in the resultant drink. This does not make them wrong or bad, it just means that they don't have the same qualities or benefits as a pure juice.

One of the greatest values of pure juices, is that they can be absorbed almost instantly by your body. Any fiber in a juice/drink will slow this process of absorption down as the body will then have to go into digestive mode. These juices are incredibly "nutrient dense".

HOW ARE JUICES USED?

Juices can be used in several ways. They can be used: as pleasurable delicious drinks, as a liquid vitamin and mineral supplement, to help prevent and protect against ill health, to help recover from certain ailments, as a meal replacement when dieting, or they can be used as the foundation of a juice fast.

I have been running supported juice fasts since 2000 for groups, individuals and even by phone/skype. Juice fasts are incredibly powerful and valuable things to do to create large shifts in your health and well being. If you are inspired by the practise of juicing, then I would encourage you to try juice fasting for 1-5 days. This book is not aimed at teaching you how to juice fast per se but it will give you the tools with which to explore the experience of short term juice fasts.

If you want to fast for longer or to do a deeper form of juice fasting detox then I would suggest that you contact me or another skilled and experienced fasting professional or detox retreat company. These types of fast can invoke healing crises and detox reactions so are best done with experienced support so that you can detox safely. Some retreats are listed at the back of this book.

Certain juices are really helpful for specific imbalances and illnesses but I do not go into those details in this particular book. For general good health it is more useful to consume a varied range of fruits, vegetables and juices, so I encourage you to get into the juice variety habit.

JUICES VS SMOOTHIES

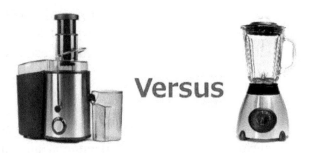

Many people seem to get the two of these drinks confused, so I am going to clearly define the difference between them. Juices are very different from smoothies – they are not better, they just have different qualities and values.

A juice is made in a juicer – centrifugal, press, masticator or auger. A smoothie is made in a blender.

Far more fruits or vegetables are used to make a juice because the fiber is removed. Therefore there are far more natural micro nutrients (vitamins, minerals, trace minerals, phyto-nutrients, enzymes) in a juice.

Less fruits and vegetables are needed to make the same quantity of smoothie because the fiber is still in the drink. Therefore there are less micro nutrients. However, there is fiber, which is beneficial for good health too. In smoothies you have the advantage that you can also add: various superfoods, fruits and vegetables that don't juice easily (bananas, avocados etc.) or nuts and seeds. These can all provide different and useful nutrients than those available in pure juices.

THE BENEFITS OF JUICING

Regular juicing can make an awesome difference to your energy, health and vitality. This has been verified many times over by thousands of research studies done in the last few decades.

A high consumption of fruits and vegetables has been associated with reductions in: heart disease, certain cancers, senility and diabetes. These are some of the main chronic diseases that have seen an increase in the last 50 years and which we have been struggling to effectively treat (in terms of reversal) with modern western medicine.

In some ways it is possible to regard fruits and vegetables as "Nature's pharmacy" because so much good can come from their consumption. In fact Hippocrates who is often cited as being the father of modern medicine was well known for saying "Let food be thy medicine and medicine be thy food," so this isn't new news at all.

5 FRUITS AND VEGETABLES PER DAY???

At the end of the 20th century the governments of the UK and USA began giving public health advice to people to try and include at least 5 portions of fruits and vegetables per day in their diet. I actually met one of the researchers who had been involved in correlating all of the research on the impact of increased fruit and vegetable intake on health, in the UK.

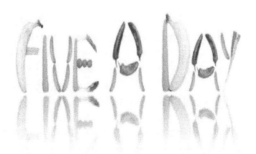

What I found fascinating was that based on the evidence that they had found, they had originally wanted to recommend that the UK government advised people to have at least 10 portions of fruits and vegetables per day for the most beneficial impact. However, in their research they had discovered that there were large sections of the UK population that were not even consuming one portion of fruits and vegetables per week!

As a result, it was deemed more sensible to recommend consuming 5 portions to start with and then over time to increase this recommendation. I have noticed recently that already in certain places, 7 portions are being recommended.

When you make your own fresh juice each day, you are easily consuming the minimum of 5 portions of fruits and vegetables per day.

It must be noted that some of the benefits of increased fruit and vegetable consumption are due to the increased consumption of fiber in the diet. Obviously, if you are juicing, you have removed the fiber, so it will not be beneficial on that level. It is therefore important that you are consuming lots of fruits and vegetables in your regular diet too.

You may also find that some fruits and vegetables when juiced, create a pulp that is still useful and could potentially be consumed as part of your other food intake e.g. courgette/zucchini, soft berries, etc. (Note: many pulps are not great though, as they are too fibrous and lacking in flavor or nutritional value – you may have to experiment to see whether it is worth using particular pulps.)

MICRO NUTRIENT SUPERHIGHWAY

The amazing thing about fresh, pure juices is that they are absolutely packed with lots of very valuable nutrients that can be quickly and easily absorbed and used by your body. They are like the perfect, natural multi vitamin and mineral liquid supplement boost for your health and energy. Actually, they are better than that because the form that these nutrients are in is highly bioavailable (easy for the body to use in its present form) whereas many supplements are not.

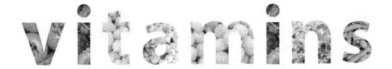

Your body does not have to become involved with the process of breaking down and digesting the juices (because in effect, they are pre-digested), it does not have to waste its own energy to do so (we require a surprisingly large amount of our daily energy just to digest food).

The stomach is a highly acid environment that can actually reduce the amount of some useful nutrients available, the longer that food stays there. As long as you are consuming your juices on their own, on an empty stomach, they do not have to stay in the stomach for long and therefore the nutrients will be assimilated by your body. In fact, the nutrients from any juice that was consumed on an empty stomach can be in your blood stream 15 minutes after drinking your juice.

The main nutrients that your body will be flooded with when drinking juices are: vitamins (A, B1, B2, B3, B5, B6, Folate, C, E and K), minerals, trace minerals, enzymes and chlorophyll. Juices also provide lots of flavonoids and phyto-nutrients (plant chemicals that have beneficial protective and healing qualities). The antioxidants found in juices are very powerful and effective at clearing free radicals from the body. There are also carbohydrates and even a limited amount of amino acids (proteins) which can be found in juices too.

This is living food in its most potent form. The dense nutrient intake that comes from regular juicing not only helps to keep you healthy and protect you from certain common diseases but

17

also can quickly have positive effects on your skin, hair, eyes, mental acuity, fat ratio, muscle tone and energy levels. Not bad for a drink that can easily be made at home with minimal effort and a fairly low cost! If someone in the food and drink or the pharmaceutical industries was able to create a substance that could do even a quarter of what fresh juices can do, they would make a mega fortune!

Detoxification

Another great thing that juices are really helpful with is supporting our body's natural detoxification processes. Our modern environment (air, water, food, personal care products) all have a lot of chemicals in them that are toxic to our bodies. Also the natural processes of metabolism in our bodies create toxins and waste products. These are processed and cleared by our bodies on a continuous basis but particularly at times when we are not involved in the digestive process such as overnight and first thing in the morning before we eat (or break-fast).

Having a juice instead of eating can extend these digestive breaks so that our bodies can keep repairing and regenerating themselves for longer periods of time.

Also the many nutrients and the high quality of natural water that are found in juices are really helpful for supporting and enhancing our body's abilities to cleanse themselves.

Many people are actually chronically dehydrated without knowing it. This inhibits both the natural detoxification processes as well as the normal functioning of the body. Regular juicing provides a fantastic source of electrolyte full water which will help the body rehydrate effectively.

It's Also A Time Saver

It is quite funny how many people have told me that they don't have time to juice because I often juice to save myself time as the process is pretty quick and easy once you get used to it. Generally, it is possible to go through the whole juicing process (preparation, juicing, cleaning and drinking) in 10-15 minutes! So if I want a nutritious snack or meal replacement quickly then making a juice is ideal.

THE SECRET OF BECOMING A JUICER IS BEING WELL PREPARED

Well actually it's not the only secret but it is an important part of the process. To this end, the next couple of chapters will provide you with the knowledge that you need to set up your juicing space with all of the right equipment.

CHAPTER 2. CHOOSING THE RIGHT JUICER FOR YOU

If you do not have a juicer of your own yet, understanding the differences between the various juicers will be really helpful and will enable you to choose whichever juicer is most suitable and useful for you.

If you do already have a juicer, this information may help you to understand the pros and cons of that juicer, as well as help you to choose a better one, if and when you are ready to upgrade or replace your present juicer.

THE LOW BUDGET JUICER

The lowest budget juicer is of course a citrus press. These are very limited in their use, as they can only be used on citrus fruits (oranges, lemons, limes, grapefruits, clementine, tangerines, mandarins, etc.) or with pomegranates. However, they are really good at what they do and are better than the other juicers for these particular fruits. It is therefore, useful to own one of these as part of your juicing kit.

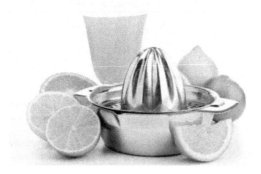

Citrus presses can be hand powered or electric. For most people hand powered will suffice but if you are likely to regularly do large quantities of citrus fruits or if your wrists and forearms aren't so strong, then you may find an electric one more useful.

CENTRIFUGAL JUICERS

The main lower cost juicer and in fact the most common one is the centrifugal juicer. This has a high speed spinning bowl of fine metal mesh and a base with small blades on it. Although these are not the best quality juicers they can be very useful as starter juicers because for anyone who is just trying out juicing, it is not necessary to spend a lot of money.

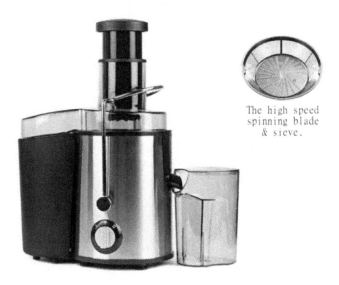

The high speed spinning blade & sieve.

So I often recommend that people start with one of these and then once they have felt the benefits and become excited and enthusiastic about juicing (or when their centrifugal juicer stops working), then they can move on to a much better juicer.

PROS: they are easy to find and buy, they are generally not very expensive (often under $50-$150 or £30-£100), they can be great starter juicers, they tend to be quite fast.

CONS: they do not tend to last a long time, they have a low yield and produce a lower quantity of juice per kilo of fruit and veg compared to the other juicers, because of the high speed that

21

they rotate at, they heat up the juice at the point of extraction and therefore damage and reduce some of the nutrients, they are unable to re-juice pulp from very soft fruits and vegetables that could otherwise have more juice extracted, juices are prone to separation, they are not very good at juicing green leafy vegetables, grasses or herbs, they can be noisy, they can be difficult to clean (this varies between makes).

THE CHAMPION JUICER– A MASTICATOR

This juicer is in a category all of its own because it's way of juicing is different to the other types of juicers. It has a spindle with rows of fine metal teeth that shred fruits and vegetables to turn them into juice which then passes through a fine mesh.

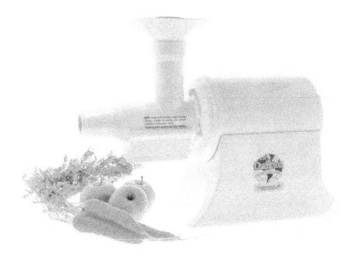

These juicers are incredibly well made having been originally designed in the 1950s when products were still built to last! The design has been altered very little since then because it is so reliable. It has a 10 year guarantee but my first Champion juicer lasted for 24 years (and the first 12 years of its life were spent in a busy café and juice bar in London, followed by the next 12 years where it was being used regularly for making juices on group detox retreats, as well as for my own juices)!

The Champion does still run at quite a fast speed but it is slower than the centrifugal juicers and therefore creates higher quality, more nutrient full juices. It is also more efficient than the centrifugal juicers, so it creates a drier pulp and more juice.

It is also far more versatile. The Champion juicer can juice green leafy vegetables (these need to be introduced alternately with harder fruits and vegetables for best effect) and it can also produce frozen fruit ice cream (made by using just frozen fruit), nut butters (made by adding nuts or seeds and oil) and there is also an optional grain attachment for milling grain!

PROS: they are very efficient, reliable and very long lasting, they produce a good quantity and quality of juice, they are really quick and easy to clean, it is possible to extract more juice from the pulp of very soft fruits and vegetables by feeding it through the juicer multiple times.

CONS: They are quite heavy (the price of having a decent motor), they are not good at juicing fine green leaf plants like wheatgrass.

COLD PRESS JUICERS - SINGLE AND DOUBLE AUGER JUICERS – THE CRUSHERS

These juicers tend to produce the highest quality of juice because they work by slowly crushing the fruits and vegetables.

A cold press juicer will produce about 35% more juice than a centrifugal juicer. It will also produce juices with about 60% more vitamin A and 45% more vitamin C. They are however much slower and can be quite bulky.

Like the Champion juicer, they can also make frozen fruit ice cream and nut butters. Some of them can even make fresh pasta! The frozen fruit ice creams by the way, are delicious and a fantastic alternative to normal sugar-laden shop ice creams.

Kids and adults love them. This multipurpose functionality can make them more useful in the kitchen, especially if you are interested in exploring more healthy homemade food options.

TYPES OF COLD PRESS JUICER

There are many types and manufacturers of cold press juicers, so I will just summarize some of the main ones. Basic cold press juicers include the Samson 6 in 1, the Matstone, the Omega and the Oscar. The vertical ones – Hurom juicer and Kuvings silent juicer. The top of the range ones – Green Power, Green Star and Super Angel.

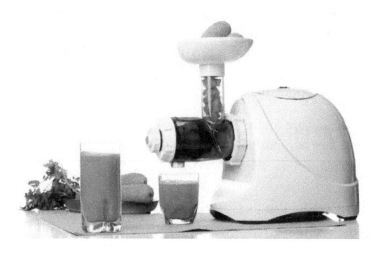

PROS: they produce the highest quality juices, they can easily juice leafy green vegetables and the likes of wheatgrass, the Hurom and the Kuvings juicers don't take up much kitchen space, juices tend to last longer because there are more enzymes left in the juices, they tend to be fairly quiet, juices last longer because of higher enzyme count, less separation of juices, it is possible to extract more juice from the pulp of very soft fruits and vegetables by feeding it through these juicers again.

CONS: juicing can be quite slow (although for just 1 or 2 glasses of juice, this isn't a big deal), juicing preparation is also slower as the fruits and vegetables need to be cut into smaller pieces, sometimes these juicers are not so good with soft watery fruits like melons, some of these juicers are quite large and therefore can take up a lot of kitchen space (Green Power, Green Star, etc.), they can be harder to clean, they are more expensive. The upright juicers like the Hurom and the Kuvings actually seem to allow a lot of fine pulp to get into the juice too.

THE RIGHT JUICER FOR YOU

So which is the best juicer for you? – The one that you have or are able to get now and will use!

If you are wary of making a larger investment yet or unable to spend much money on a juicer at the moment, then get a simple centrifugal juicer. Develop a regular juicing habit with this and notice how awesome you feel. When your machine breaks down or when you get to a point in time that you want to try making better quality juices or juices with green leafy vegetables then move on to a Champion or a cold press juicer.

WHERE TO BUY A JUICER

Juicers can be found in most kitchen or department stores these days, although these are often just the cheaper centrifugal ranges of juicers. If you are starting with one of these, then this can be an easy option.

If you want a wider choice and higher quality juicers to choose from then often the easiest option is searching on the internet. I would recommend the Vitality Juicer websites which can make this process much easier, as they research some of the best deals that are presently available on the internet and have the different types of juicers in easily laid out categories. They can be found at:

www.vitalityjuicers.com in the USA

www.vitalityjuicers.co.uk in the UK

CHAPTER 3. THE JUICER'S KITCHEN KIT

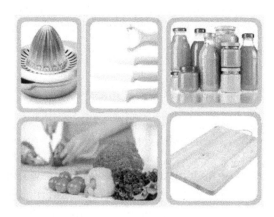

So now that you have or know which the best juicer for you is, you have the most important part of your juicing kit. Here are some other tools and useful items that you will find really helpful for making juices and maintaining a regular juicing habit.

A CITRUS PRESS

One of these simple juicers is really useful and very affordable. Adding lemon or lime to juices can help bring out their flavors or take the bitterness out of certain juices.

GOOD QUALITY KNIVES

It is always easier to have sharp, good quality chef's knives to work with, as they make the process much faster. If you don't know how to use professional knives safely, then I would suggest that you either learn (no doubt there are YouTube videos) or use less sharp knives.

A GOOD QUALITY PEELER

A good peeler is really helpful for quickly peeling non organic vegetables.

CUTTING BOARDS

I recommend that you have at least 2 cutting boards in your kitchen. One board should only be used for cutting pungent vegetables such as garlic and onions, as well as chili when cooking or juicing (don't ever try juicing onions – yuck!!). The other should be used for all other fruits and vegetables. The reason for this is that pungent flavors and spices can be transferred via the cutting board. There are few things that can make fresh melons or other fruit juices taste as bad as the lingering after taste of garlic or onion!!!

VEGIWASH OR APPLE CIDER VINEGAR

These can be useful to add to water and wash any non-organic fruits or vegetables that you use. They help to remove some of the pesticides and herbicides.

A POURING JUG

My preference are the Pyrex glass ones. Some juicers actually come with jugs. The important thing is that it pours easily, as it can be very frustrating to lose half of your delicious fresh juice to the table in a pouring accident.

STORAGE BOTTLES

Although generally it is best to drink your fresh juice straight away, there may be occasions and reasons for storing your juice in the fridge. For this purpose I would recommend sealable glass bottles or BPA free plastic bottles (so that chemicals don't get into the juice). Alternatively, glass jars can be very useful for storing small amounts of juice in the fridge. These need to be airtight to reduce the amount and speed of oxygenation.

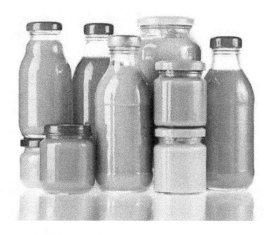

Don't store your juices in open jugs in the fridge, as these will allow fast oxygenation and deterioration of your juice.

BIODEGRADABLE PULP BAGS

Many juicers have a pulp collecting tub and some require that you use a bowl or container of your own. Either way, it is useful to have some of these bags as they can reduce the cleaning up process.

If you have a compost in your garden you are very lucky because juicing pulp turns into fantastic soil once it has been composted.

A GOOD SCRUBBING BRUSH AND WASHING UP SPONGE

These are just for cleaning your juicer and juicing equipment.

AND NOW FOR THE GOLDEN NUGGETS

So that is all of the equipment taken care of. If you already have it, you can start making juices but before you do I highly recommend that you read the following chapter about tips and tricks that will simplify the juicing process. These are the golden nuggets of juicing wisdom that can transform you from being someone who owns a juicer (which is stored in a cupboard somewhere) into someone who is a juicer!

Chapter 4. Tips And Tricks To Make Regular Juicing Much Easier

I was quite tempted to call this chapter "Tips and Tricks to Make Daily Juicing Much Easier". However, I know all too well how the pressure and expectation of thinking that you have to make a juice every day or else you will fail, is almost definitely going to get in your way or make you give up.

And it is not that you have to have a fresh juice every day to be doing it right. I don't juice every day, although I do miss it on the days that I don't manage to have a fresh juice and I certainly feel better on all of the days that I do have fresh juices. It is more useful to juice as much as you are able to and to really pay attention to how different you feel on the days when you do juice and the days that you don't.

The tips and tricks that I am going to suggest in this chapter are all habits that will help you to make juicing easy, enjoyable and something to be enthusiastic about.

Tips

1) Pay great attention to how you feel after you have had a fresh juice.

Juices can give us a much greater sense of health, energy and vitality but it is not enough to just know the theory of this, as it will have limited impact on you and the choices that you make. If however, you really pay close attention to how you feel on the days that you juice and even on your general health and well-being overtime, it will become a true bodily felt knowing and an integrated wisdom that is very likely to inspire you to juice regularly.

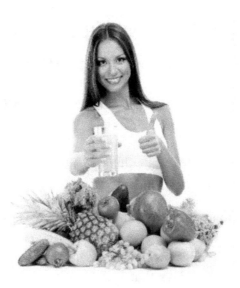

You may even notice over time that different chronic health problems that have been nagging you for years diminish or disappear. Flooding your system on a regular basis with the nutrients that it needs to maintain and repair itself can start to have noticeable effects on your body's ability to function well.

2) Always, always, always rinse and wash your juicer as soon as you have finished creating your juice!

Of course you can sip it with appreciation beforehand but make sure that the juicer is cleaned ASAP. A juicer is easiest to clean at the moment that you stop using it. The longer that you leave it, the more effort that it can be to clean it, so get into the habit of doing it straight away. For some of the juicers, this process may be as simple as rinsing it under a running tap. Others may require a bit of scrubbing with a brush but either way, it's much easier when done immediately.

3) Buy your fruits and vegetables in bulk so that you always have plenty to choose from and use.

It can also be good to plan ahead a bit when going out to buy your fruit and veg or when ordering it online. If you know that there are some new juice recipes that you want to try, add the ingredients to your shopping list ahead of time.

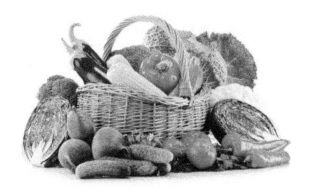

Apart from buying fruits and vegetables from local stores and supermarkets there also some other great bulk shopping options. Many places have organic veggie box schemes where you can order online and have them delivered to your house. Also you could check out farmers markets. And of course one of the best ways, if you are so inclined and have the ability, is to grow your own!

4) **When using fruits that go very soft upon being ripe, use them just before they become ripe.**

Especially for some of the soft fruits like kiwi fruit, it is best to use fruits that are still fairly hard, as these will juice more easily

5) **If using organic vegetables, do not peel them first.**

The skins of many fruits and vegetables contain a lot of nutrients, so it is good to juice them too. Conversely, the skins of many non-organic fruits and vegetables contain a lot of pesticides and are therefore best peeled.

6) **Wash non organic fruits and vegetables.**

If you are using non organic produce it can be useful to wash it first using either a proprietary fruit and vegetable washing agent such as "veggie-wash" or a bowl of water with a tablespoon of apple cider vinegar. At the very least, wash them in water. If you wash your non organic veg when you first bring it into the house, you do not have to be bothered with washing it every time that you want to make a juice.

7) Avoid having excessively sweet juices.

If you are using fruits and vegetables that are very sweet, then make the juice less sweet by either watering it down or using unsweet vegetables as well. This will reduce the likelihood of you spiking you blood sugar and therefore will keep your energy levels more balanced.

If you have diabetes or blood sugar problems then you are best off just creating juices predominantly with vegetables and avoiding using many of the vegetables that are very sweet like pineapple.

8) Try replacing your coffee hit with a natural juice energy boost.

It is a much healthier option – better energy with no come down, no side effects, no blood sugar imbalances and no addiction!

9) Do not bother to store juice made in a centrifugal juicer.

Because of the heat and the high oxygenation involved in the process of juicing with a centrifugal juicer, the juice is prone to losing its nutrient value quite quickly, therefore it is best to drink it as soon as you have made it, or certainly within a couple of hours of having made it at most.

10) Use Biodegradable compost bags to collect your juicing pulp as this will reduce your clean up time.

11) Some fruits or vegetables can go through the juicer several times to extract more juice from them.

This is particularly true of soft fruits like raspberries, strawberries, melons, etc. but also some vegetables like zucchinis (courgettes) or cucumbers (yes I know that these are actually fruits too but in the normal world most people think of them as vegetables). You can tell which juice pulps can be re juiced because it is not very dry at all.

The Champion juicer especially but also some of the cold press juicers are able to extract more juice from the resultant pulp if it is collected and fed back through the juicer several times. The pulp will become drier and less in quantity each time that it goes through.

Unfortunately, this will not work with a centrifugal juicer.

12) Use the freshest fruits and vegetables that you can.

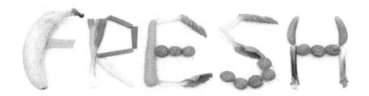

The fresher the fruits or vegetables are, the more nutrients are still in them.

13) Some fruits do not juice

Fruits like bananas, soft papaya, soft mango and avocado will not juice in most juicers. Instead, it is better to use these fruits in smoothies.

14) Do not juice potatoes

It is the only vegetable that I can think of that is not good for juicing. (Sweet potatoes are fine). It's also worth mentioning that you should never juice the green leafy tops of carrots, just in case you have fresh carrots with the tops still on.

15) Drink Juices on an empty stomach

Your body will be able to absorb the most nutrients from a juice if you consume it on an empty stomach. The optimal time to drink a juice is at least ½ hour before consuming any other foods and 2 hours after any other foods. Having said that, it may not be optimal at other times but it will still be great!

16) Keep discarded vegetable stems from your cooking.

Things like broccoli stems that many people throw away whilst cooking are actually fantastic for juicing, so put them in your fridge instead of the compost/bin and use them in your next juice.

17) Drink slowly and savor

To get the most nutrients and help you become a real juice lover, it is best to drink slowly and with awareness. In the naturopathic tradition we suggest that you should chew your juices and drink your food (drinking food is only possible if you have chewed it really thoroughly first). These habits really support your body's digestion.

18) When using a non-centrifugal juicer, cut celery into small pieces.

Celery and similarly stringy vegetables (fennel, parsley and some of the green leafy vegetables as well as pineapple core) are best cut into 4cm (1½ inch) lengths to stop the fibers binding around the juicer's spindles or augers. This can block the juicer and stress the motor. Juice them last.

19) If making a juice with citrus fruit in it, use a citrus press to juice the citrus part of the juice.

20) **Prepare all of the fruits and vegetables first.**

If you wash and chop up all of the ingredients first and then feed them all into the juicer in one go, it will be a faster process.

21) **If you are planning to have a morning juice but have limited time, then do your preparation the night before.**

It can be much easier if your fruits and vegetables are all sitting ready in your fridge when you wake up in the morning.

22) **Explore and be creative with your juice recipes.**

I really encourage you to try lots of different juice recipes from this book (these will give you a great foundation in what fruits and veggies combine well) and also create new ones. Being creative keeps the process fun and alive.

TRICKS

1) **If it is feasible in your kitchen, always keep your juicer out on a kitchen counter surface where it is clearly visible and not in the way.**

This tip is to stop you becoming just a juicer owner but rather be a juicing enthusiast instead. As they say "out of sight, out of mind" and this is very true of juicing machines. I can't tell you how many people that I have worked with on my detox retreats who have told me that they own juicers but upon further questioning it has turned out that the juicer is in the back of a cupboard somewhere and has not seen the light of day for years!

So keep you juicer out in clear view where it is easily accessible. This will remind you to make juices. It will make the process of setting up your juicer that much quicker and easier. It will also potentially be a talking point for visiting friends and family who may already be interested to know why you look so healthy and vibrant.

2) Try a "30 Day Juicing Challenge"

Decide to juice at least once every day for 30 days. It will require a bit of organizing and preparing with having enough fruits and vegetables but it will be great preparation and practice for you. You might even want to encourage some of your friends to join you, to keep mega motivated. The value of such a challenge is that being committed to this practice you will quickly develop the habits that enable you to juice regularly. Plus you are very likely to clearly experience some of the amazing benefits that consistent juicing brings. Both of these consequences will support you to juice much more regularly in your normal life.

3) Keep a Juice Recipe Journal

When experimenting and inventing juices (or even if you are trying out new recipes that you discover and really like), it can be invaluable to have your own juice recipe journal to keep a record of them. This can be a simple notebook or you could use a book that has been specifically designed for this, such as "My Favorite Juice Recipes Book" which can be found in various book sellers and at: www.journaleasy.com/health-cooking-journals

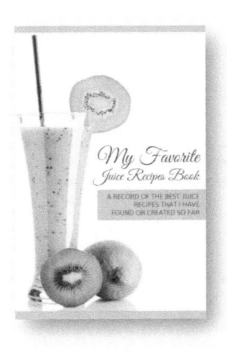

On each page of your journal it will be useful to keep the name of the juice (or to make one up that you will remember) for easy reference, a list of the fruits or vegetables needed to make it and perhaps a mark out of 10, to remind you how much you liked it.

In this way, you will be able to create a collection of your own favorite juices in a relatively short period of time.

4) **Treat your friends and family to fresh juices.**

It can be great to make juices for friends when they visit or for your family, because not only will you be helping them in that moment but you may even inspire them to take up the habit of making fresh juices for themselves. Having more inspired and healthy people in your environment will make it even easier for you to keep up the fantastic habit of regular juicing.

Simple, generous and inspiring actions like this can end up rippling outwards and encourage lots of people. As regular

37

juicing can have such a profound effect on people's health, happiness and wellbeing, it can be great to know that you have had been such a positive influence on your community.

5) **Have occasional "Juice Days"**

It can be great to occasionally only consume juices for a day. No food, just juice. Such days can be really valuable, as they give your body a complete rest from the digestive process, so that it has a chance to cleanse and detox, whilst the same time you are giving it a mega dose of nutrients to boost your vitality.

If you are the sporty type then you might really benefit from combining your juice day with time at the gym, running cycling, swimming or participating in whatever form of exercise that you really enjoy.

If you are the more chilled out type, then you might like to combine this with time at a spa, having a massage, a gentle walk in the countryside, a hot bath with aromatherapy oils, time on the sofa with a good book or whatever nurturing pastimes that you really enjoy (but probably don't make time for in your normal life).

Of course you can also spend the day using a combination of the above two approaches. And don't think that you need to spend this day on your own. You could also get together with a group of like-minded friends and share the experience to make it more fun.

One word of warning though, if your normal diet and lifestyle isn't great, you may get some detox symptoms such as headaches, the first few times that you spend the day on just juices. Don't worry and try not to reach for the paracetamol, as it is just your body cleansing itself and it will pass and get easier.

STORING JUICES AND MAKING THEM LAST LONGER

The best time to drink a freshly made juice is when it is fresh! The longer the juice is left before being consumed, the more the useful nutrients (vitamins, enzymes and phyto-nutrients) degrade and diminish.

However, it is often impractical to have your juicer with you whenever you want to have a juice. You may also want to reduce the amount of time that you are spending juicing but want to have more than one juice in the day. It is therefore useful to have ways to store juices as well as have strategies and techniques for having fresh juices when away from home.

The easiest strategy is to get someone else to make a fresh juice for you. This is sometimes possible if you are near one of the many new juice bars or cafes that make fresh juices. If you are lucky (or have inspired them) you may be visiting friends or family who juice regularly and you might be able to join them when they are juicing.

I do not however, encourage you to buy a juice in a carton from a shop in these circumstances though, as these drinks lack many nutrients and are often loaded with sugar or sweeteners and other additives.

Often it will be up to you and your own self sufficiency to be prepared with a juice of your own. There are a couple of ways that you can do this.

Once you have made a juice it is very important to keep it cool or to make it cool, so put it in a bottle* and into the fridge straight away. Better than this, it would be really useful to put the juice in a freezer for 15 minutes and then to put it in the fridge. This reduces the temperature of the juice very quickly and then keeps it at this temperature, which will greatly slow down the rate at which the juice nutrients diminish.

* When you need to store fresh juices, it is best to do this in a sealed glass or BPA free plastic bottle or in a glass jar. Fill this container as close to the top as you can to reduce oxygenation.

To have your cooled juice later in the day at work or wherever it is that you intend to drink it, you can keep it in that bottle and put it in a fridge, if there is one there. Alternatively, you could transport it in a thermos flask to maintain it at its cooled temperature.

The other thing that you can do is add a teaspoon of vitamin C powder to your juice, which will slow down the oxidation and deterioration. This will impact the flavor though and it is still recommended to store it in a refrigerator too.

It is always best to drink a fresh juice on the same day that it was made, even when it has been preserved in this way.

As mentioned in the Tips section of this chapter, it is not advisable to try storing juices that have been made in a centrifugal juicer, as they lose their nutrient value quite quickly. You can of course use the techniques outlined above to store these juices if you wish and it is really necessary but do not store them for long and know that they are at their optimum the moment after they have been made.

N.B.

Avoid Grapefruit if you are on some medications!

Grapefruit interferes with your Liver's ability to process toxins. Although some pharmaceuticals can be useful they are nearly all toxic to the body and need to be cleared by the liver. Many medications are designed to be dealt with by the body in a certain way which may not happen if you consume grapefruit. This is not true for all medications but it is worth you checking the small print and warnings on the information that comes with any pharmaceuticals that you might be taking.

Avoid cleaning your teeth for ½ hour after drinking sweet fruit juices.

Fruit juices can soften the enamel on the teeth, especially the more acidic or sugary ones. For this reason it is good not to brush the teeth for about 30 minutes after these juices. After that time, the enamel should have returned to its normal hardness.

ALMOST READY TO START MAKING JUICES?

If you have children who you would love to encourage to drink fresh juices, then the next chapter is for you.

If not, then feel free to skip to the following chapter which will prepare you for diving into the juice recipes.

Chapter 5. Tips To Inspire Children To Love Fresh Juices

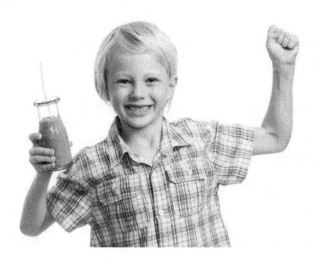

A lot of the people that I have worked with have been really keen to get their children to start drinking juices too but have not been able to get them to do so.

The first things to do is to inspire and show them (this works for friends and family too, who will want to know why you are looking so healthy and vibrant). Children learn by watching what their parents and the people around them do. If they see their parents drinking and enjoying juices regularly, they are likely to want to try them too.

Secondly, make juices a treat! What makes a treat a treat? Answer: the label that we give it.

Having lived in numerous countries around the world, I have seen many different foods and activities being offered as treats (including such unlikely things as fresh chilies in Indonesia) and they are always responded to by children in the same way, because they have been described as being special. Unfortunately, in the modern western world, treats have become synonymous with unhealthy and addictive sugar packed sweets! But it doesn't have to be that way. It is just about what you have taught them is a special food, so make your treats fantastic, vitamin packed, fresh juices.

Incidentally, this practice works just as well for our own inner child (the aspect of your own young self that still lives on as part of your psyche and emotional body). It is also helpful to get into the practice of rewarding yourself with a vibrant fresh juice at times.

Thirdly, do not make excessively sweet juices for your children, as this can help get them hooked into the addictive sugar cycle. To make juices less sweet, you can add bland but water-full fruits and veggies to the juice, such as cucumber. It can also be useful to add water to the juices (maybe make them 1/3 or ¼ water).

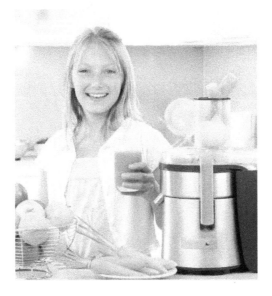

Fourthly, involve your children in the creative process. When kids are actually making the juices themselves you can be surprised at the unexpected fruits and vegetables that they are willing to put in the juice and drink afterwards. Naturally, it will be good to supervise this process, to make sure that they do not create any horrendous, "put you off for life" juices made from the likes of onions and potatoes but generally you will find that they will choose the ingredients intelligently and in fact may introduce some great new recipes into your repertoire. Keep a record of them in your Juice Recipe Journal.

Finally, here is a great way to make juices in the summer fun – make ice pops from fresh juices! Kids love ice pops in the summer and frozen juice ones go down really well (I even know of a mother who used to put spirulina in ice pops for her kids and they loved them!!!) All you need are some ice pop molds and a freezer. Easy!

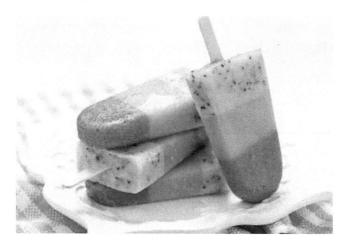

CHAPTER 6. HOW TO USE THE JUICE RECIPES

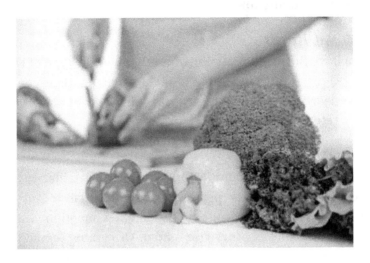

The recipes that you will find in this book are designed to give you a sense of the incredible range and types of juices that you can make. If you love them, then keep making them. If you aren't so keen, then try another one.

Once you have started to get an idea of what fruits and vegetables go together well and how to make different types of juices, I would like to encourage you to start experimenting and inventing your own juices. Having a sense of fun and adventure in your juice making is one of the things that will keep you interested in juicing regularly. Keep records of your successful juice experiments in your Juicing Journal.

Know now that some of your experiments are probably not going to turn out very well but when that happens you can learn not to mix those veggies in those sorts of quantities again. Often, you can also recover a disaster juice by adding extra apple or carrots or lemon.

RAW

It may seem obvious but I have known people who have attempted to juice the likes of cooked beetroots, so I just want to clearly state that **everything that you attempt to juice needs to be raw and uncooked**.

PERSONAL NOTES

If you have the printed version of this book or the type of Kindle or e-reader that it is possible to make notes on, then you may want to write a comment or give the juice a score out of 10 for future reference to yourself.

QUANTITIES

These recipes have quantities of fruits and vegetables to make an 8-12oz glass for one person which is all that you actually need as a serving. All fruits and vegetables mentioned are of medium size unless otherwise stated. Of course, the size and liquid content of a fruit or vegetable can vary greatly, so this is only a guideline.

If the juice is very sugary, it is advisable to water it down.

HOW TO PREPARE FRUITS AND VEGETABLES

There are many different types of fruits and vegetables that you can use whilst juicing and they all have to be prepared in different ways that may even vary between juicers. To be able to discover and learn the best, easiest and most nutritionally useful ways to prepare your fruits and vegetables, I wrote a fruit and vegetable preparation guide which you can download and print out for quick reference in the kitchen.

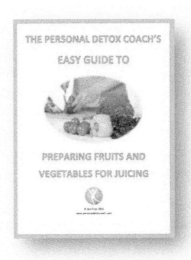

To get your free guide, your tips, more juice recipes and your updates go to:

http://www.personaldetoxcoach.com/JuiceHabitBookSign

TASTE

Taste varies from person to person so some people will love some recipes and others will not. Sometimes our taste is influenced by what our normal diet is like and if it is normally full of processed foods, then we are likely to be drawn to the sweet juices and to not enjoy the vegetable juices so much to start off with. However, I would encourage those of you who find themselves in this position to keep trying the green juices and the less sweet ones because as your body becomes more alkaline and less sugar addicted you will be likely to find that your tastes change too.

SPICES

There are a couple of spices that I am going to recommend that you use in some juices – ginger and chili! When using ginger it is possible to have a rough idea of how spicy it is by quantity, although this can vary.

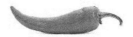

Chilies however, can vary massively in how strong they are. For this reason I would encourage you to err on the cautious and minimalist side. Add a small amount to the main juice and then test it. If it requires more, you can add a bit more. It is good to remember that you can always add a bit more but if you add too much you can't take it out!

Your aim when you are using these spices is to bring their flavor into the juice without overpowering the other flavors within the juice.

The warmth that these spices bring to juices can also be really valuable as it makes juices more desirable in the cold winter months. From a Chinese dietary perspective, fresh juices are very Yin and therefore cooling, by their nature. Generally in the winter months we are naturally drawn to more Yang warming foods. Having ginger or chili in your juices sometimes will make them more appealing and warming to your body when it is cold.

Whilst I am on the subject of ingredients to use with care, it is worth me mentioning garlic too. Garlic is wonderful because of its antibiotic, antifungal and blood cleansing properties but it is also incredibly strong in its raw form in juices.

If you ever feel inclined to add it to one of your vegetable juices because you want to try it or you love garlic or because you have a cold that you want to clear more quickly, then I would suggest that you use a quarter of a clove at the most per glass of juice.

It has a very strong, overpowering flavor and should be used carefully. In this book I only suggest the use of garlic in a couple of recipes just so that you can get a sense of how it can influence the flavor. If you really love garlic and you don't have any social engagements then you could always try using a greater quantity!

Herbs

Some of the recipes include herbs which can introduce really delightful flavors to your juices. Only use fresh herbs though, as dried herbs will not juice and lack taste.

It can be difficult to juice herbs in centrifugal juicers though, as much of the leaves can be sent straight to the pulp container. Try mixing the herbs with the other fruits or vegetables as much as possible whilst feeding them into the juicer as this will at least help some of the leaves to be juiced.

Use Organic If Possible

As much as you are able, use organic fruits and vegetables. You will soon discover that these are normally much more flavor-full. More importantly, they have far fewer chemicals on them that can cause a toxic build up in your body over time.

Pesticides and herbicides that are used in modern farming are poisonous by their very nature and although these might be in small quantities, their constant consumption has been traced as a cause of various types of cancer and other diseases. Bearing in mind that these are designed specifically to be poisonous to various life forms it is not so surprising that they are harmful to us too.

Organic fruits and vegetables have also often been found to have higher nutrient content. One of our main goals with juicing is to get more nutrients in our bodies, so it makes great sense to use the ingredients which are naturally bursting with more nutrients.

So Now That You Are Fully Prepared........

IT'S JUICING TIME!

CHAPTER 7. FRUIT CENTERED JUICE RECIPES

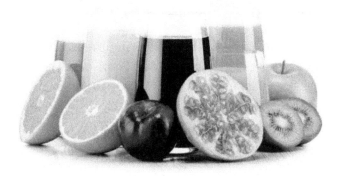

This chapter is focused on fruit juices which are cleansing and light. For most people who have a normal western diet which is laden with sugars and sweeteners, these are the juices that they will be drawn to first. Many people are often addicted to sugar and high GI (Glycaemic Index) foods that turn into sugar quickly (wheat products and other such simple carbs are a good example), without being aware that they are addicted. The long term effect of such a diet is extremely detrimental to health and is a great part of the cause of the obesity and diabetes epidemics that we are presently seeing in the world.

Ideally, it will be good to move away from the high sugar foods by consuming natural sugars in juices and less processed foods, this can be a great way of starting to make that shift. However, it is also important not to transfer your sugar addiction to very sweet juices. If you do find that you have an excessive desire just for sweet juices, then I would recommend that you aim to use the less sweet recipes that include less sweet vegetables (bearing in mind that some root vegetables are actually very sweet too e.g. carrots, parsnips, beetroot, etc). Adding cucumber is ideal for this. Also adding water to your juices can be helpful.

As you get used to and inspired by the vital and alive taste of fresh juices, then I would encourage you to shift to drinking more vegetable juices which are even more effective at nourishing and rebuilding your body on a cellular level.

As I stated, fruit Juices by their very nature are very cleansing and can be a great way to start a day. Some of these juices I will suggest as breakfast juices because after fasting overnight this is our optimum natural detoxification and cleansing time. In actual fact, they can be drunk at any point in the day.

MORNING GLORY

This can be a fabulous way to start the day with "get up and go" or as a really refreshing midday, summer drink.

INGREDIENTS:
Quarter of a small Watermelon

4 fresh Mint leaves

COMMENTS:
Remove the watermelon skin and use the red center, including the watermelon pips.

If you are using a centrifugal juicer, it will not be able to juice the mint leaves easily, so double the quantity of leaves and try and feed the leaves in mixed with the melon.

If you are using an organic watermelon, an even more nutritious version of this juice can be made by using the skin of the watermelon too.

PERSONAL NOTES:

PINK BREAKFAST

This is a delicious and sharp drink to start the day with.

INGREDIENTS:
½ a Pink Grapefruit

1 cup of fresh Raspberries

COMMENTS:
Add the raspberries to the juicer first. As they are quite pulpy, with non-centrifugal juicers it can be worth feeding the pulp back through the juicer several times to get more juice out of them.

The grapefruit can be juiced using a citrus press or by removing the peel and putting it into your juicer.

It is important to use pink grapefruit because it has a lower GI (sugar content) than yellow grapefruit. As mentioned in the tips section, take care with grapefruit if you are on medications.

PERSONAL NOTES:

WARM SUNRISE

This is another great juice to start the day with and because of the ginger it can be enjoyable even on cold winter days.

INGREDIENTS:
½ Gala Melon

2 Oranges

½ cm (¼ inch) Ginger

COMMENTS:
The Melon can be re-fed through non-centrifugal juicers several times.

The oranges are easiest to juice with a citrus press.

I am suggesting ½ cm of ginger but the appropriate amount will depend on the strength of the ginger, so juice the ginger first and see how the flavor is at the end. Add more if necessary.

PERSONAL NOTES:

PINEAPPLE REFRESHER

This is a very nice refreshing juice. Normally pineapple can make juices very sweet but the cucumber softens the flavor and reduces the sugar content.

INGREDIENTS:

1/3 medium Pineapple

1/3 Cucumber

½ Lemon

COMMENTS:

You will need to cut off the skin from the pineapple. The pineapple and the cucumber go straight into your juicer.

The easiest way to juice the lemon is with a citrus press.

In the winter, you might prefer the following recipe - Ginger-Pineapple Ale Juice which is similar but warmer.

PERSONAL NOTES:

GINGER-PINEAPPLE ALE JUICE

This is a delicious warming juice which can even have a fizz if you choose.

INGREDIENTS:

1/3 medium Pineapple

¼ Cucumber

1 Apple

1cm (½ inch) slice of Lemon

Optional sparkling water

COMMENTS:

Cut off the skin of the pineapple and then put all of the ingredients through the juicer. For this recipe, the slice of lemon actually goes through the juicer with the peel still on.

If you would like the juice to be even more like a ginger ale, then you can add natural sparkling spring water to it.

PERSONAL NOTES:

STRAWBERRY PUNCH

This is a delicious and refreshing summer juice.

INGREDIENTS:
3 x Apples

¼ Cucumber

1 cup of Strawberries

COMMENTS:
Juice the strawberries first. If you are not using a centrifugal juicer, you can re-feed the strawberry pulp through your juicer a few times to get more juice from them. Then juice the other ingredients too.

PERSONAL NOTES:

CHRISTMAS SURPRISE

Who would have thought about having a juice at Christmas? Well now you have this healthy option, although you can also delight in its flavors at any time of year. This juice, as the name implies, was inspired by the traditional festive fruits that Christmas is celebrated with in the northern hemisphere.

INGREDIENTS:
2 handfuls of fresh Cranberries

8 x Satsumas or Tangerines

COMMENTS:
Juice the Cranberries first then either juice the satsumas/tangerines with a citrus press or peel them and juice them in your main juicer.

If you want to give it an even more festive flavor, you could even add a ¼ teaspoon of cinnamon powder!

PERSONAL NOTES:

CHERRY FRESH

This is a nice summer juice that can be made into a sparkling drink too.

INGREDIENTS:
2 x Apples

2 cups of pitted fresh Cherries

½ Lemon

COMMENTS:
Put apples and cherries through the juicer. Use the citrus press for the lemon.

This is another juice that it can be nice to add natural sparkling spring water to for that added refreshing fizz effect.

PERSONAL NOTES:

ANTI-OXIDANT BLAST

This is a great one for keeping your immune system up.

INGREDIENTS:

2 x Apples

1 large handful of Grapes with seeds

1 cup of Blueberries

¼ Lemon

COMMENTS:

Do use grapes that have seeds because there is a chemical in the seeds (oligomericproanthocyanadin) that acts as a very powerful antioxidant. Also it's best to use organic grapes because non organic ones have very high pesticide residues.

It is always helpful to juice the berries first and if not using a centrifugal juicer, you will find that you can re-feed them through the juicer several times. Then juice the apples.

The lemon can be done with a citrus press.

PERSONAL NOTES:

Summer Bright

This is a very refreshing juice that is not as overly sweet as orange juices are sometimes.

INGREDIENTS:
½ Cucumber

2 Oranges

4 Fresh Mint leaves

COMMENTS:
The oranges can be juiced with a citrus press.

In non-centrifugal juicers you can re-juice the cucumber pulp.

If you are using a centrifugal juicer, it will not be able to juice the mint leaves easily, so double the quantity of leaves and try and feed the leaves in mixed with the cucumber.

PERSONAL NOTES:

MAGICAL POMMES

I named this one magical pommes because apples are called pommes in French and I had never noticed the similarity of name or fruit before. Somehow pomegranates are like magical apples.

INGREDIENTS:
3 x Apples

1 x Pomegranate

COMMENTS:
A genius alternative way to juicing pomegranates with the citrus press is to cut the pomegranate in half, then turn the halves upside down and lightly tap them with a hammer. This loosens all of the beautiful fruit jewels inside which can then easily be removed, collected and put through your normal juicer.

Juice the pomegranate first and then the apples

PERSONAL NOTES:

APPLE, PEAR AND GINGER

The name says it all. A nice warming juice.

INGREDIENTS:
2 x Apples

2 x Pears

½ cm (¼ inch) Ginger

COMMENTS:
It is useful to use pears that are still hard and firm when juicing.

If you intend to store this juice, then add ½ squeezed lemon to it too, as this will stop it oxidizing and turning brown so quickly.

PERSONAL NOTES:

Kiwi Cooler

This is a refreshing vibrant juice.

INGREDIENTS:

4 x Kiwis

2 x Apples

¼ Cucumber

COMMENTS:

Peel the kiwis first (I once had a juice made with whole kiwi fruits at a juice bar in Portugal and I assure you that a hairy juice is not a pleasant experience!) Use hard, almost ripe kiwi fruits as they are easier to juice.

Cucumber and kiwi fruits can be re-fed into non-centrifugal juicers.

PERSONAL NOTES:

PINEAPPLE SURPRISE

About

INGREDIENTS:
1/3 Pineapple

1 x Apple

¼ Cucumber

½ Lemon

A cup of Parsley

COMMENTS:
Remove pineapple skin before juicing. Pineapple and cucumber can be re-fed through non-centrifugal juicers.

Push the parsley through the juicer using the apple. If using a centrifugal juicer, then you may need to use 2 cups of parsley.

PERSONAL NOTES:

Old Favorite – Apple, Carrot, Ginger

This is one of the simplest and enjoyable fruit and veg juices to make. It is one that people often get stuck on as the main one they make. For this reason, I am including it for you to try if you have not done so yet but don't get stuck on it – there are so many other great juices to try too.

INGREDIENTS:
2 x Apples

4 x medium Carrots

½ cm (¼ inch) Ginger

COMMENTS:
An easy juice. Just feed the ingredients into the juicer!

If the carrots are not organic, then peel them first.

PERSONAL NOTES:

ARABIAN NIGHT

This is a very refreshing and cooling summer drink that has some of the classic flavors that are prominent in the Middle East.

INGREDIENTS:
2 x Apples

¼ Cucumber

6 fresh Mint leaves

¼ Lemon

COMMENTS:
The cucumber, apple and mint can be re-fed into non-centrifugal juicers.

If you are using a centrifugal juicer, it will not be able to juice the mint leaves easily, so double the quantity of leaves and try and feed the leaves in mixed with the apple chunks.

Use a citrus press for the lemon.

PERSONAL NOTES:

LEMON MERINGUE PIE JUICE

Sure that sounds like a bizarre name for a juice but when you taste it you will totally understand why it is so aptly named.

INGREDIENTS:
4 x Apples

¼ Lemon or 2cm (¾ inch) slice (whole)

COMMENTS:
Put the lemon with its rind through your normal juicer with the apples.

A quick and easy juice

PERSONAL NOTES:

Autumn Fresh

This juice is great to make late summer or autumn when there are lots of fresh blackberries out and the orchards are full of apples and pears.

INGREDIENTS:

2 x Apples

2 x Pears

2 cups of fresh Blackberries

COMMENTS:

All fruits can go straight into your juicer. Put the Blackberries in first. If you are not using a centrifugal juicer then the pulp can be re-fed through your juicer.

PERSONAL NOTES:

PEACH PASSION

A fruity & fresh drink

INGREDIENTS:
3 x Peaches

1 x Apple

5 x mint leaves

Squeeze of Lemon

COMMENTS:
Stone the Peaches before feeding into your juicer (I know it may seem obvious but I just want to stop any mishaps happening).

PERSONAL NOTES:

APPLE-BEET-PINE-CUC

An unusual rich juice

INGREDIENTS:
1 x Apple

½ Beetroot

¼ Pineapple

¼ Cucumber

COMMENTS:
The pineapple and cucumber can be re-fed into non-centrifugal juicers.

PERSONAL NOTES:

SWEET AND SOUR

This juice can have a great juxtaposition of tastes with the sweet pineapple and the bitter cranberries that together create something quite unexpected.

INGREDIENTS:
1/3 Pineapple

1 cup of Cranberries

½ Lemon or Lime

COMMENTS:
Remove pineapple skin. Squeeze lemon or lime with citrus press. Try it and see.

PERSONAL NOTES:

THE DIGESTER

This juice's ingredients are all helpful for digestion, so it can be a great juice to make if you suffer from indigestion. It is also a really nice juice to have even if you don't have digestive problems.

INGREDIENTS:
1/3 Pineapple

2 x Kiwi Fruits

1 cm (½ inch) Ginger

8-10 fresh Mint leaves

½ Lemon

COMMENTS:
Remove skin from pineapple and kiwis. Mix mint with these and the ginger as you juice. Juice the lemon with a citrus press.

PERSONAL NOTES:

RED ORANGE

This has a similar juxtaposition of flavors as the previous juice. It looks like it should be a strong beetroot juice but actually tastes strongly orangey.

INGREDIENTS:
3 Oranges

½ Beetroot

COMMENTS:
Juice oranges on a juice press and beetroot in a juicer, then combine.

PERSONAL NOTES:

SUNSET SOOTHER

This is a delicious juice that is great to try whenever you see pomegranates in the shops. It makes a stunningly colorful juice and even though it's titled a sunset juice, it really can be drunk at any time.

INGREDIENTS:
2 Pomegranates

2 Oranges

COMMENTS:
Both the oranges and the pomegranates are most easily juiced by using a citrus press.

PERSONAL NOTES:

Mojito

A very refreshing juice that is slightly reminiscent of the infamous Cuban Mojito cocktail.

Ingredients:

½ Cucumber

1 x Pear

1 handful of fresh mint leaves

Comments:

An awesome summer picnic or garden drink. Add crushed ice for the full mojito-like experience.

Personal Notes:

CHAPTER 8. VEGETABLE BASED JUICE RECIPES

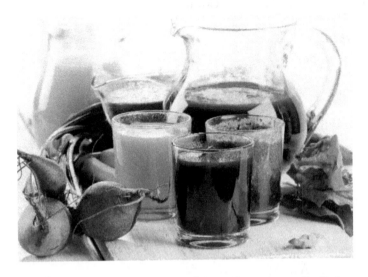

The vegetable juices have a tonifying, cleansing, alkalizing and building effect on the body and your cells. These types of juices are more useful for your daily consumption and will give you a longer more sustained energy boost than the fruit based juices.

The green leafy vegetables are particularly good to use. These are plants like spinach, watercress, cabbage, kale, rocket, romaine lettuce, parsley, etc. as the high levels of nutrients like chlorophyll and magnesium are very useful for the body. However, when you make a green juice, try not to make it with more than about 25% of its volume being composed of green leaf juice, as it is very strong and can ruin the taste.

Beetroot is another very strong vegetable that you shouldn't use too much of. Generally I recommend not creating a juice where beetroot is more than a 1/3 of the juice volume.

Whenever you make a green juice that does not taste great, you can often fix it by adding extra carrots or apple or by adding lemon juice. So if you are experimenting with creating your own juices, don't give up straight away. Some of my favorite juices were resuscitated 'failures'.

PEPPERISE

This can be a refreshing morning juice.

INGREDIENTS:
½ Yellow Pepper

½ Red Pepper

4 x Carrots

COMMENTS:
Remove tops of carrots and seeds of peppers, then juice.

PERSONAL NOTES:

"Lunch"

I named this one lunch because it is what I just made myself for my lunch! It was totally inspired by what fresh vegetables I had in my fridge and it was delicious. I encourage you to try this juice and as you get used to what fruits and veggies combine well, to start experimenting with what is in your fridge today too!

Ingredients:
4 x Carrots

1 x Broccoli stem

1 x Apple

5 x small pink Radishes

¼ Fennel bulb

½ Green Pepper

2 handfuls of fresh Spinach

½ Lemon

Comments:
Lemon should be squeezed. The rest go in the juicer.

Personal Notes:

GAZPACHO

This juice is inspired by the Spanish cold soup of the same name and has the same ingredients

INGREDIENTS:
4 x Tomatoes

½ Green Pepper

¼ Cucumber

¼ of a Garlic clove

4 Basil leaves

COMMENTS:
Adjust the quantity of garlic as needed. Be aware that real tomato juice has a tendency to separate and look quite watery and foamy. Just keep stirring it. Basil will not juice easily with a centrifugal juicer so add 2 x the amount and mix it with the veggies as you juice them.

This does create a very wet pulp that can be re-fed through non-centrifugal juicers or it can actually be used as a cold gazpacho soup.

PERSONAL NOTES:

LIVER TONIC

Here are some great vegetables that support your liver function. They are useful in general life and also for those of you who have occasional nights of excess partying.

INGREDIENTS:
3 x Carrots

½ Beetroot

1 x stick Celery

½ Apple

COMMENTS:
A really great basic veggie juice that you can add extra green leafy vegetables to.

PERSONAL NOTES:

Parsnip and Pear

A surprisingly sweet and unexpected flavor.

INGREDIENTS:
2 x hard Pears

2 x Parsnips

1 x stick of Celery

¼ Cucumber

COMMENTS:
Add water if it is too sweet.

PERSONAL NOTES:

FENNEL FUN

An almost bizarrely tropical taste!

INGREDIENTS:
½ Fennel bulb

¼ Cucumber

¼ Pineapple

½ Lime

COMMENTS:
Remove pineapple skin. Juice lime on a citrus press.

PERSONAL NOTES:

Sweet Potato Surprise

If you had not considered using sweet potatoes in juices before, here is your chance to try it.

INGREDIENTS:
½ Sweet Potato

3 x Carrots

½ Beetroot

COMMENTS:
This is a sweet juice, so water down if necessary

PERSONAL NOTES:

THE REAL V8

The V8 drink that can be bought in tins and cartons has some great vegetables in it but they have been cooked and processed!? This is a real version of that juice and is far better.

INGREDIENTS:
4 x Tomatoes

2 x sticks of Celery

¼ Beetroot

1 handful Watercress

1 handful of Spinach

¼ Lettuce

2 x Carrots

1 cup fresh Parsley

COMMENTS:
You may need to keep stirring this to stop it separating.

PERSONAL NOTES:

THAI CARROTS

It's not a Thai recipe at all but it does have a hint of that delicious cuisine.

INGREDIENTS:
6 x Carrots

1 cup of fresh Coriander leaves (Cilantro)

¼ Lime or Lemon

COMMENTS:
Chop the coriander/cilantro up into 3cm or 1 inch lengths. Feed alternately with the carrots into the juicer.

If using a centrifugal juicer do not cut the coriander/cilantro and use twice as much.

Use the citrus press for the lemon/lime.

PERSONAL NOTES:

Green Joy

This is a very energy-full drink. You will notice that the zucchini/courgette gives it a pleasantly creamy taste.

INGREDIENTS:
1 x green Apple

1 x Courgette/Zucchini

1 x Broccoli stem

3 x handfuls of Spinach

1 cup of Parsley

COMMENTS:
For non-centrifugal juicers, the zucchini/courgette can be re-fed through the juicer several times to extract more juice.

PERSONAL NOTES:

THE REFRESHER

This is one of my favorite summer juices.

INGREDIENTS:
½ Cucumber

1 x Apple

2 sticks of Celery

¼ or ½ Fennel

½ Lemon

COMMENTS:
Cut celery into smaller chunks. Re-feed cucumber through juicer if non-centrifugal. Juice lemon on a citrus press.

PERSONAL NOTES:

ORANGE GREENS

This juice is a good example of how the strong flavor of oranges can cut through the normal green flavors to create something quite different.

INGREDIENTS:
2 x Oranges

½ yellow Pepper

1 x Broccoli stalk

3 handfuls of Spinach or

3 handfuls of Kale

COMMENTS:
Juice the oranges on a citrus press, the rest in a juicer.

PERSONAL NOTES:

THE COLD CURE

For those who love garlic or are fighting off a cold. Lots of vitamin C and Zinc in this one too.

INGREDIENTS:

1 Red Pepper

1 x Courgette/Zucchini

2 x Carrots

5 x large Kale leaves

1 x Broccoli stem or 4 florets

1 handful of Parsley

½ clove of Garlic

½ cm (¼ inch) Ginger or ½ cm (¼ inch) Hot Chili Pepper

½ squeezed Lemon

COMMENTS:

If using chili in this recipe use a small amount ½ way through the process and taste to get a sense of how strong that particular chili is and whether to add more or not. If you are keen you can have ginger + chili but have some tissues ready.

PERSONAL NOTES:

ROOT JUICE

This is great to show you how sweet the root vegetables are.

INGREDIENTS:
½ Sweet Potato

2 x Parsnips

2 x Carrots

¼ Beetroot

5 large Kale leaves

COMMENTS:
If the root vegetables are not organic then peel them first. If they are organic you can whizz them straight through the juicer - another advantage of eating organic foods!

PERSONAL NOTES:

Vampire's Delight

So named because of its rich color and flavor.

INGREDIENTS:
½ Beetroot

2 x Carrots

1 x Apple

½ Fennel bulb

1 handful of Spinach

COMMENTS:
An easy and quick juice.

PERSONAL NOTES:

SPRING FRESH

A very refreshing and light juice. Ideal in the spring, summer or whenever you like!

INGREDIENTS:
1 x Apple

¼ Cucumber

¼ Fennel bulb

1 cup fresh Peas

4 x Mint leaves

COMMENTS:
If using a centrifugal juicer you may need 2 x as much mint.

PERSONAL NOTES:

CELERIUM

A simple veggie juice.

INGREDIENTS:
3 sticks of Celery

½ Cucumber

1 x Tomato

1 handful of Coriander

COMMENTS:
If using a centrifugal juicer you may need 2-3 x as much coriander to get a sense of its flavor.

PERSONAL NOTES:

HAPPY HALLOWEEN

This is a great one for having in October when we are suddenly treated to loads of pumpkins in the shops.

INGREDIENTS:
3-5 cups of cut and cubed Pumpkin

2 x Carrots

1 x Apple

1 ¼ cm (or ½ inch) Chili

COMMENTS:
Use chili with care because it is difficult to be accurate with this measurement as chilies can vary massively in how hot they are. It's better to use less to start with or use a chili that you know is fairly mild.

PERSONAL NOTES:

Salad In A Glass

A very different way to enjoy a salad.

Ingredients:
¼ Cucumber

3 x Tomatoes

½ Lettuce

½ Pepper (any color)

1 cup of fresh Parsley

½ squeezed Lemon

Comments:
This one may separate so be prepared to keep stirring it. Mix the parsley between other vegetables to help it juice better.

Personal Notes:

GREEN SPICE

Fresh watercress adds a lovely spicy flavor to juices and is also very nutritious.

INGREDIENTS:
2 sticks of Celery

1 x Carrots

1 x green Apple

¼ Cucumber

2 x handfuls of Watercress

COMMENTS:
It will be helpful to cut the watercress into shorter lengths (5 cm or 2 inches) if you are using a non-centrifugal juicer.

PERSONAL NOTES:

Beet Vite

Often people throw away the green tops of fresh beetroots but they are actually really packed with nutrients and great to use in juices.

INGREDIENTS:
½ Beetroot + the Beet Greens

2 x Carrots

1 x Apple

1 cm or ¼ inch Ginger

COMMENTS:
I recommend that whenever you are able to get fresh beetroot with the leaves that you definitely keep the leaves for juicing.

PERSONAL NOTES:

THE COLD BUSTER

If you notice the first signs of a cold coming in (sniffly nose, tickly throat) and make this juice, you can stop it ever coming in or certainly speed it through your system. This is an alternative more spicy juice to the "Cold Cure" recipe.

INGREDIENTS:
1 ½ cm (½ inch) Ginger

1 x Chili Pepper

½ Garlic clove

8cm (3 inches) Mooli Radish

½ Red Pepper

1 Apple

2 handfuls of chopped Kale

COMMENTS:
This is a very hot and spicy drink, so you may have to adjust the quantities to what you personally can handle (although the hotter that you can handle, the more effective it is). You might be surprised how tasty it is!

PERSONAL NOTES:

MUSTARD MAGIC

A mustard tinged fresh veggie juice

INGREDIENTS:
 3 x Carrots

2 x Celery Sticks

¼ Cucumber

1 or 2 Mustard Greens leaves

COMMENTS:
 Adjust the Mustard Greens leaf quantity – it should only be enough to create a mustardy overtone.

PERSONAL NOTES:

FRESH AND FAST

This is a light, quick and easy green juice, for a refreshing energy boost at any time of day.

INGREDIENTS:
½ Cucumber

½ Green Pepper

1 x Apple

¼ Lemon squeezed

COMMENTS:
If not using a centrifugal juicer you might want to refeed the cucumber pulp through a couple of times to extract more juice.

PERSONAL NOTES:

SHAOLIN BREAKFAST

Another light green juice with some interesting flavor tones.

INGREDIENTS:
2 x Celery sticks

½ Cucumber

7 x Bok Choy leaves

¼ Fennel bulb

½ Apple

COMMENTS:
A squeeze of lemon juice can also be added to this to bring extra flavors through.

PERSONAL NOTES:

CHARDELICIOUS

A very tasty green leafy juice

INGREDIENTS:
7 x Chard leaves

2 x Pears

1 cm or ¼ inch Ginger (optional)

¼ squeezed Lemon

COMMENTS:
Chard leaves may need to be chopped into smaller lengths.

PERSONAL NOTES:

PUMPKIN PUNCH

An interesting juice with lots of Vitamin A which is an important antioxidant and is particularly useful for maintaining the health of your skin and eyes.

INGREDIENTS:

3 cups of Pumpkin

2 x Carrots

1 x Broccoli stem

7 x Romaine Lettuce leaves

½ Apple

COMMENTS:

The pumpkin does not actually have to be cut up to fit in a cup – the "3 cups" suggestion is just so that you have an idea of the right quantity. Remove the pumpkin's skin if it is not organic.

PERSONAL NOTES:

PARSLEY PASSION

Parsley is a very nutritious plant but rarely used in juices. It can also mask the flavor and odor of garlic, so there is an option of adding a bit of garlic to this juice for its health benefits and flavor, if you would like to.

INGREDIENTS:
3 cups of chopped Parsley

2 x Carrots

2 x Broccoli stems

4 x small Radishes

½ Apple

(Optional - ¼ clove Garlic)

COMMENTS:
You may wish to adjust the optional garlic quantity to your particular taste or 'social needs'.

PERSONAL NOTES:

POPEYE'S REVENGE

A rich green and nutritious pick-me-up juice.

INGREDIENTS:
The equivalent of 8 cups of Spinach

½ Cucumber

¼ Pineapple

Squeeze of Lemon

COMMENTS:
The spinach does not actually have to be cut up to fit in a cup – the "8 cups" suggestion is just so that you have an idea of the right quantity

PERSONAL NOTES:

CHAPTER 9. FAQs

Will juicing regularly help me lose weight? Juicing regularly can be very helpful for losing weight. Useful strategies for losing weight with the aid of juicing include replacing one meal per day with a vegetable juice, as well as juice fasting for a few days.

Of course, this needs to be part of an overall action plan to be effective. Such a plan should include removing sugar and other unhealthy processed foods from the diet, stopping snacking, eating moderate size portions at meal times and regular exercise.

How long will it take me to feel the benefits of regular juicing? Normally when someone makes a dietary change it is recommended that they allow 3 months to be aware of the changes that have occurred. However, with regular juicing, people are often aware of the differences that are being made within a week.

Are there any juices or fruits/vegetables that it could be harmful if I had too much of them? I would certainly recommend that you don't have too much high sugar fruit juices as these can either maintain unhelpful sugar addictions or disturb blood sugar levels. A vegetable like beetroot is very strong and should only be used in combination with other vegetables, being a maximum of a third of the content. Also, be aware that if you do make a juice with beetroot it is likely to have a coloring effect that you may notice later on in the toilet (so nothing to panic about). Generally however, you will be fine with all other fruits and vegetables and their juices.

When is the best time to have a juice? Whenever it is easiest for you to make it. It doesn't really matter when you have a juice when you start, so I would recommend that you start making them whenever it is easiest for you to do so in the day. However, if you have your juices instead of breakfast on some mornings you will be extending your natural overnight fasting and cleansing cycle, which would certainly be beneficial.

Also, it is helpful to have your juice on an empty stomach i.e. at least ½ hour before any other food and 2 hours after any food. This will give your body the optimum level of nutrients.

Can I use juices as a meal replacement? Yes, juices can make very good meal replacements. Whether it is for losing weight or for convenience of time, I would recommend that you replace a meal with a vegetable based juice. If doing this on a regular basis it is best to just replace one meal in this way and to still have two good healthy meals as well.

Is it OK for me to just live on juices for a week or more? Would it be safe? This book is really aimed at supporting people to drink fresh juices more regularly in their normal daily life rather than coach people through extended juice fasting.

Extended juice fasts can be very beneficial but unless you have a great deal of experience with fasting, I would suggest that you find an experienced and qualified practitioner or a fasting retreat center that can support you going through a longer fast. Generally, juice fasting on your own for up to 5 days should be fine. When people fast for longer periods they are more likely to face detox symptoms, healing crises or signs that they need to stop fasting. A professional can support you through this or tell you to stop if it is necessary.

The other benefit of a fully supported juice fast and detox is that a team of good professionals can help you go through a much deeper process, often on an emotional, mental and spiritual level as well as on the physical level. As a result, these supported fasts are much more powerful.

There are also some people and certain health conditions that would not be suitable for juice fasting. Pregnant women are not encouraged to juice fast, rather it would be much better for them to supplement their diets with fresh juices for the extra nutrients that are so valuable for the creation of a healthy baby. Diabetics have to juice fast carefully, so it is useful to have expert support. People with eating disorders should either avoid fasting or just do so with support.

Can I use the juice pulp for anything? It seems such a waste to throw it away. If you have a non-centrifugal juicer some of the more wet pulps can be re-fed into the juicer and juiced several times to extract more juice out.

You could perhaps use some of the fiber in some cooking but I wouldn't recommend using much because the pulp can be quite tasteless and very fiber-full. Many years ago I bought a juicer for my Mother who is of the WW2 generation and therefore very careful not to be at all wasteful. She couldn't bear the idea of throwing away all of that good vegetable matter after juicing and so for a while was in the habit of making rather bland and very fibrous soups with it. After a time, even she realized that it wasn't worth trying to do.

If you have your own garden, a great use for the juice pulp is in your compost. Mixed with occasional sheets of cardboard and inhabited by a good supply of worms, the pulp makes incredible compost over a few months

How long does it take to make a juice? Generally the whole process of preparing, juicing, cleaning up and drinking a juice only takes 10-15 minutes.

Are any of the juices good for any particular illnesses and ailments? Juices can definitely be used to support you in recovering from & coping with certain illnesses and imbalances. However, in this book I have not focused on using juices in this refined manner (apart from "The Cold Cure" and "The Cold Basher"). Rather my goal has been to encourage you to drink any and many juices on a regular basis. Consuming a broad

111

variety of juices will be incredibly helpful for boosting your immune system and providing a multitude of nutrients for maintaining a great level of health.

I will be publishing future books that are focused more on using specific juices to help with certain ailments, so if you are interested in this way of juicing then sign up here to be notified when they are available: **CLICK HERE**

APPENDIX – JUICE RECIPE NAMES

Fruit Centered Juice Recipes

Breakfast Juices

Morning Glory

Pink Breakfast

Warm Sunrise

Pineapple Refresher

Anytime Fruit Juices

Ginger-Pineapple Ale Juice

Strawberry Punch

Christmas Surprise

Cherry Fresh

Anti-Oxidant Blast

Summer Bright

Magical Pommes

Apple, Pear and Ginger

Kiwi Cooler

Pineapple Surprise

Old Favorite – Apple, Carrot, Ginger

Arabian Night

Lemon Meringue Pie Juice

Autumn Fresh

Peach Passion

Apple-Beet-Pine-Cuc

Green Spice

Beet Vite

The Cold Buster

Mustard Magic

Fresh And Fast

Shaolin Breakfast

Chardelicious

Pumpkin Punch

Parsley Passion

Popeye's Revenge

About The Author

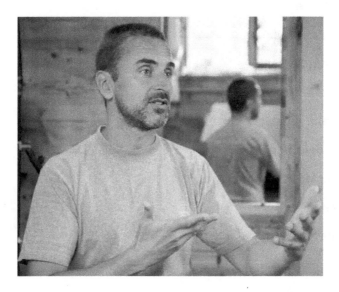

Jem Friar is a Naturopathic Consultant and a Personal Detox Coach, as well as being trained in many forms of bodywork. He has run juice fasts and Detox retreats since 2000 and has been a Detox Manager at Detox International, Spa Samui and Moinhos Velhos, as well as having his own very successful UK based detox company "Vitality Detox Retreats". In 2007, he was filmed as part of the detox team in the "Spa of Embarrassing Illnesses 3" TV series and also in the "Spa of Weight Loss for Life" TV series.

Jem is well known for the private one-on-one bespoke retreats that he runs for clients around the world, as "The Personal Detox Coach". These retreats are more personalized and are for people who want that direct deep level of support but are unable to go on group retreats (perhaps because they have small children/farm animals/businesses to run) or because they prefer the privacy of such a retreat due to celebrity status, etc.

To connect with Jem and other people in the juicing community, you can like and join his Facebook page at: https://www.facebook.com/PersonalDetoxCoach

Learn more about Jem at: wwww.personaldetoxcoach.com

AND DON'T FORGET YOUR GIFT

As I said at the start of the book I would like to offer you this quick reference guide to preparing any and all of the fruits and vegetables that you might want and need to put in your juicer to help you with your new juicing habit.

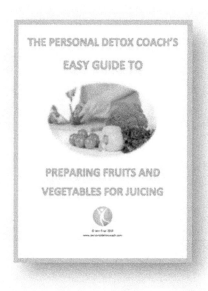

I will also inform you about any updates to this kindle book (more tips and recipes) or other juicing and health books in the Personal Detox Coach's Simple Guide to Healthy Living Series as they are released, as well as occasionally send you more scrumptious juice recipes to keep you inspired.

To get your free guide, your tips, more juice recipes and your updates go to:
http://www.personaldetoxcoach.com/JuiceHabitBookSign

OTHER BOOKS BY JEM FRIAR

The Kindle Version

Firstly, you might be interested to know that this book is available in an ebook form and is available through Amazon's Kindle MatchBook scheme at a reduced price. Sometimes it is just really helpful and nice to have book's in an easily portable and accessible form as well.

"THE HEART MEDITATION – a meditation to change your world" by Jem Friar

The Juicing Book series

Jem has a series of juicing books that will be available on Amazon or by direct order shortly. A couple of these will be available for free if you have signed up to receive the free fruit and vegetable preparation guide and the latest book news. These books are more focused on the health benefits of particular juices, the value of simple juices, juice fasting and intermittent fasting.

Journal Easy's Blank Recipe Books

These are designed to inspire and encourage you to keep records of any great recipes that you find as well as to experiment and create new recipes. These books are really useful and can be found on Amazon and or at: www.JournalEasy.com

My Favorite Juice Recipes

My Favorite Smoothie Recipes

119

My Favorite Vegetarian Recipes

My Favorite Vegan Recipes

My Favorite Raw Food Recipes

Juicing And Detox Retreats

If you are interested in participating in a fully held and supported juice fasting detox retreat, then you might want to have a look at:

www.personaldetoxcoach.com
- for 1 on 1 coaching and retreats with Jem.

www.detox-international.com
- for 7 day group retreats in Spain.

www.vitalitydetoxretreats.com
- for 4 and 7 day small group retreats in the UK.

One Last Thing...

If you enjoyed this book or found it useful I'd be very grateful if you'd post a short review on the site through which you bought this book. This will help other potential readers know how helpful this book will be for them too.

Also I try to read all the reviews personally so that I can get your feedback and make my books even better.

Thanks again for your support!

CPSIA information can be obtained
at www.ICGtesting.com
Printed in the USA
BVHW041211240221
600993BV00013B/321